FIVE MINUTES TO DE-STRESS

How to Kick Stress and Anxiety
in 5 Minutes or Less
Using Any of These 60 Easy Techniques

S.K. Sands

TABLE OF CONTENTS

INTRODUCTION

Okay, first the bad news: stress is not good.

Well, actually, it *can* be good. If you notice the approach of a galloping, rage-filled rhino while you're enjoying a walk in the Serengeti, you want stress to kick in to get you the hell out of there. Thank you, stress. But we all know, barring any run-ins with raging rhinos, most everyday stress is bad.

How bad? For starters, it can kill you. It can damage the heart, cause you to gain weight, raise your risk of disease and erupt in a hairy mole on the side of your nose (okay, maybe not that last one).

Stress comes from those everyday pressures we feel in life, a current situation upsetting our normal balance that makes us frustrated, angry or nervous. Anxiety is stress that continues after the situation is gone, adding a dose of fear or apprehension, and often a feeling of impending doom, in the mix.

It's easy to see that reducing stress is a top-notch way to improve your physical, mental and emotional health. And who doesn't need that?

We'll be exploring a number of remedies for getting the upper hand on that emotional intruder. About sixty of them, in fact.

Let's take a look.

REMEDIES

We all get stressed, of course. That's life. But that doesn't mean we can't stomp our foot, stick out our bottom lip and take control. Just who is in charge here, anyway? (You are—honest.)

Five minutes is all it takes to have a significant impact on how you feel and how you cope with life's little (and sometimes big) irritations, frustrations, annoyances—and fears. To kick them to the curb. To say *Hit the road, Jack* with a meaningful thrust of the thumb over your shoulder. Yeah, you got this.

In only five minutes, you can de-stress in any one of several ways. The first is something you're likely already doing.

Chapter One

BREATHING

Good old breathing.

Aside from keeping us alive, breathing can not only increase energy and boost alertness, but special techniques can also soothe the nerves. One of the main advantages is they can be done anytime, anywhere.

When we get rattled, our breath tends to become short and shallow, pushing our stress level ever higher. But focusing on breathing can cause positive effects almost immediately. As the body begins to relax, allowing emotions to level off, the heart rate begins to slow while blood pressure drops back into a healthier range. Ahhh, much better.

* * *

Breathe slowly in and out through the nose, with the exhale lasting longer than the inhale. Slow, deep breathing for just a few minutes can decrease your tension level dramatically.

* * *

Place the tip of your tongue on the roof of your mouth just behind the back of your top front teeth.

With your mouth slightly open, exhale completely while making a whooshing or sighing sound.

* * *

Close your mouth and inhale through your nose for a count of four, hold for seven and exhale for eight.

* * *

Get into a relaxed position, either lying down or sitting up.

Inhale deeply and slowly into your abdomen, feeling it move upward as it expands. It should feel similar to a balloon expanding.

At the end of the inhalation, exhale slowly and completely, allowing your abdomen to fall as you exhale. The expiration should last about twice as long as the inhalation.

Repeat a few times, focusing on your hands rising on the abdomen as you inhale and falling as you exhale.

* * *

Try to set up a special signal to yourself as a reminder to stop what you're doing to take a deep, calming breath. For example, you might touch your middle finger and thumb together on each hand—something that can be easily and privately done wherever you are. Standing in line at the grocery store, sitting down for a job interview, scraping off a wad of chewing gum—whatever you're doing, stop and take a breather.

For a guided breathing process, please see RESOURCE GUIDE at the end of the book.

Meanwhile, just keep breathing. It does wonders for your health.

Chapter Two

FOOD

Eat something—anything! (Well, maybe not *anything*.)

It's normal to become stressed and irritable when you're hungry (who, you?). Feeling stressed could indicate a drop in blood sugar. A good solution is to have a quick, healthy snack.

Actually, your diet can be the key to reducing those frazzled nerves. You might try eating more whole natural foods (the kind not found in a box): meat and fish, vegetables (especially leafy greens), fruits, nuts and seeds. The closer the food is to its natural, straight-from-Mother-Nature state, the better. In other words, finish all your veggies at dinner. Come on now.

And, yes—also a good idea to cut back on the bad favorites like candy and pastries. Which is no fun at all. But you don't need to eliminate such treats, just limit to one serving per day. You could simply replace some sweets with fruit. But a taffy apple doesn't count.

So what to eat? Let's find out.

* * *

- Toss back a handful of walnuts

  The nutrients in walnuts may reduce stress by providing mood-enhancing benefits, in addition to helping manage the impact stress has on the cardiovascular system.

- Grab a stalk of celery

  Certain nutrients in celery can have a sedative effect, so chomp on a stalk or chop some into a salad. Then relax. Maybe take a quick nap.

- Munch on cherries

  These little red gems soothe the nervous system and relieve stress.

- Crunch on lettuce

  Like celery, this popular and omnipresent veggie can have a nice sedative effect. The substance responsible is the white, milky juice you see when a stalk of the lettuce is snapped. And you thought lettuce was boring.

- Eat whole wheat bread

    Also whole-wheat pita, whole-grain cereal, pasta, and brown rice. These all rank high in the B vitamins, helping to sustain the nervous system. For a stress-fighting diet, consider getting about 60 percent of your daily calories from these sources. But when the stress is reduced, you might want to cut back a bit or you may end up with bigger problems (yeah, talking about weight gain here).

- Chew away

    Chewing gum may not be pretty, but it can be relaxing. Chomping on a stick of flavorful resin can reduce cortisol during times of stress. Plus snapping it with attitude gives you a jaunty way to take your mind off your troubles.

- Pop in a piece of chocolate

    What better way to stimulate the release of those beta endorphins, the body's feel-good drug? Okay, a banana is a good choice, too, as its potassium can also regulate blood pressure. Or how about a dark-chocolate-covered banana? Now we're talking.

- Sip a cup of hot tea.

  Seems the Brits and Japanese have had it right all along. Drinking tea can reduce stress levels and promote a calming effect. It also provides healthy antioxidants to boot. So boil some water, brew your favorite tea and take a five-minute break to relax and rejuvenate while you sip in peace. Or slurp. Go ahead. Nobody's listening.

Okay, time to head to the kitchen.

Chapter Three

ESSENTIAL OILS, HERBS AND TEAS

With these highly concentrated aromatics, it's important to use caution. In general, these oils are not indicated for use on those who are pregnant or breastfeeding, for infants or young children, people with serious medical conditions, or certain pets—especially cats.

As a general rule, it's recommended that for topical use, they be diluted in a carrier oil (e.g., almond, coconut or olive). For adults, use 3-5 drops of essential oil per teaspoon of carrier oil. Before using a new essential oil on the skin, it's a good idea to do a small patch test to check for sensitivity or skin irritation before applying to a larger area of the body.

Always check for potential interactions with medications before using any essential oil or herb.

* * *

<u>ESSENTIAL OILS</u>

Smells. Or aromas. Aromatherapy, to be exact.

Certain scents from nature can not only reduce stress, but also promote better focus and concentration.

Aromatherapy is the use of essential oils that have been extracted from plants for medicinal use. This holistic medicine has been around for over 6,000 years. Plenty of time to get it right.

The secret lies in the stimulation of the limbic system that then releases chemicals to increase feelings of relaxation and lying-on-a-warm-beach, sand-in-the-toes tranquility. Oh, yeah.

Conveniently, essential oils come in small bottles that can await you on a shelf at home or travel with you on the go. Inhale deeply of the oil that most appeals to you or dab a little on your temples for a longer-lasting effect.

Some of the best scents for stress-relief are basil, chamomile, and ylang-ylang, in addition to the following:

- Cypress

  Cypress oil is thought to have a grounding and balancing effect, soothing those tense, tight muscles while supporting localized blood flow. Altogether, these aspects can deliver a one-two punch to stress for a solid knockout.

- Rosemary

  Rosemary oil can lower cortisol levels. Along with stress relief, rosemary can also enhance mental clarity and memory. And who can't use that?

- Lavender

  Lavender oil is known for its soothing scent. It can lower your heart rate and regulate blood pressure, assisting in relaxing and acting as a sedative to reduce feelings of stress and anxiety.

  Lavender can be consumed as a tea, but it may work better by breathing in the essential oil via a diffuser.

  Another possibility is using a combination of scent and touch (touch itself has a calming effect on the body and mind) by making a massage oil. Use three to four drops of lavender to a teaspoon of carrier oil (olive, sesame or almond). Lavender is one of the few essential oils that can even be safely applied directly to the skin undiluted.

An added bonus: lavender oil seems to be beneficial in the treatment of hair loss.

Less stress and more hair. That's a win-win.

- Valerian

  One of the main uses of valerian is to cure insomnia and improve the quality of sleep. But it's also widely used to improve mood and reduce anxiety. The same properties that enable better sleep also act to reduce chemicals in the body that induce anxiety and stress. This helps rebalance the body and increase the sense of peace and calm.

  Most people take valerian as a capsule or tincture. Try consuming it close to bedtime and you may start cutting some z-z-z-z's.

  NOTE: Due to its sedative effects, check with your doctor before taking valerian. And, of course, avoid driving or using machinery for a few hours after ingesting.

Valerian shouldn't be used in combination with alcohol or by children, or women who are pregnant or breastfeeding.

For information on where to buy essential oils, see RESOURCE GUIDE at the end of this book.

* * *

HERBS

- Chamomile

    This is one of the best-known stress-reducing herbs. Used for centuries to calm frazzled nerves, it also has a mildly sedating quality and can be useful for those having difficulty sleeping due to stress. It can be brewed in a tea or taken as a supplement.

- Passionflower

    Not surprisingly, considering the name, this herb is known as an aphrodisiac in ancient Polynesian cultures. It's known for relieving high levels of anxiety. Its effects are mildly sedative. This would seem to run counter to its use as an aphrodisiac, but there it is. It can be brewed as a tea or taken as a liquid extract (up to 45 drops daily).

- Ashwagandha

  Also known as winter cherry, this herb has been used for thousands of years to soothe the agitated mind. It's known as an adaptogen, meaning it helps us 'adapt' to our environments, including the stressful ones. Take as a supplement (300 mg standardized ashwagandha once or twice a day).

- Lemon balm

  This herb can reduce stress while improving calmness and alertness. And who doesn't like to pucker up with a jolty taste of sour lemon? It can be used as an aromatic or as a supplement (300-500 mg of dried lemon balm, or 60 drops, daily).

* * *

TEAS

Brew a cup of herbal tea, then sit back, put your feet up, and sip for five minutes. (Of course, if you can manage, ten would be better. Maybe even fifteen. Or twenty. Ah, heck—take the rest of the day off.)

- Mint

    Add a few sprigs of mint to two cups of hot water; steep for 3-7 minutes. Or simply toss a few mint leaves into your summer herbal tea or garnish your dessert for a refreshing twist.

- Rosemary

    Put one teaspoon of leaves in a cup of boiling water; steep for 5-7 minutes. Can also be paired with lavender and thyme.

    NOTE: Avoid rosemary tea during pregnancy!

- Oregano

    Add three teaspoons of fresh oregano leaves or one teaspoon of dried oregano to a large cup of boiling water; steep for 5-10 minutes (the longer you steep, the stronger the flavor).

- Thyme

    Use one teaspoon of dried thyme for each cup of hot water; steep for 5-7 minutes. Strain the herbs and add honey and/or lemon, if desired.

- Basil

    Put about two tablespoons of fresh cut basil in a cup of hot water; steep for 7-10 minutes. Strain.

- Lavender

    Add one tablespoon of fresh or dried buds to a cup of boiling water; steep for 5-10 minutes.

- Lemon Balm

    Place two teaspoons of fresh or one teaspoon of dried lemon balm in a cup of boiling water; steep for 5-10 minutes.

And there you have it—oils, herbs and teas. Choose one—choose all. And enjoy.

Chapter Four

CANNABINOIDS

We've all heard of cannabis. Both CBD and THC are cannabinoids that are naturally present in the hemp plant. Most marijuana products are high in THC, which leads to the "high" felt on ingesting them. But CBD, due to its different chemical makeup, affects our brains in other ways, helping reduce stress and improve mood naturally.

In other words, CBD oil can be a great alternative for those who want to feel relaxed without getting stoned.

The existence of hemp can be found throughout recorded history. Some believe it was the first crop domesticated by our ancestors, producing food, medicine and textiles. From the mid-1800s to the mid-1900s, hemp oil was a natural part of the U.S. drugstore scene, and doctors would regularly recommend it for their patients. Cool doctors. Then came the Controlled Substances Act in 1970 and hemp was now on the naughty list.

While both are part of the Cannabis family, marijuana and CBD are obviously not the same and are used for different purposes. However, this distinction didn't stop our great leaders from getting confused and lumping all Cannabis species together, banning the whole kit and kaboodle.

Now, with hemp more difficult to obtain, Americans became deficient in cannabinoids. What the heck are those?

It turns out those are things your body needs. We all have special receptors that are part of the body's endocannabinoid system (ECS). This system is responsible for regulating certain physiological functions related to appetite, pain sensation, mood and memory. Most of these receptors are located in the brain and nervous system and are activated by cannabinoids. When the ECS is out of whack, you're more susceptible to disease and other disorders.

The ECS is affected by both endocannabinoids (cannabinoids created by the human body) and by those that are plant-sourced. Here comes CBD galloping to the rescue, binding to certain receptors related to pain and inflammation. One of these receptors stimulates serotonin production, helping to reduce stress and improve mood. Since stress and pain are often connected, cannabidiol can work to reduce both simultaneously. A two-for-one special.

Many proponents claim it can also regulate sleep patterns and improve mental health (sign me up).

BUT IS IT LEGAL?

The defining difference between marijuana and hemp is the percentage of THC present. Marijuana refers to cannabis containing higher levels of THC. Hemp refers to cannabis containing less than 0.3% THC.

While CBD Oil from industrial hemp would contain no traceable amounts of THC in the end products, please verify its legal status for consumption in your state or country.

HOW MUCH CBD OIL SHOULD YOU USE?

CBD comes in a variety of formats. In addition to the oil, it can be used in a vaporizer, as a spray or consumed in foods.

According to online sources, you might start at 2-3 milligrams per day and work your way up to 100-200 milligrams—*but please do your own research before using.* CBD oil takes a few minutes to a couple of hours to take effect, depending on your metabolism and how you take it.

Note: Data on long-term use of CBD oil is limited. While research strongly points to the positive role cannabidiol can play in treating short-term anxiety, little is known about its long-term effects. Use caution in the case of prolonged use.

Chapter Five

MUSIC AND MOVEMENT

CRANK UP THE SONGS

Music can do wonders for body and soul, putting you in a happier place instantly. So turn up the volume, shake the windows, and feel those good ... good ... good vibrations. (You're thinking of the song, aren't you?)

- Choose the memories

  Play some tunes that will trigger positive images from the past. Maybe a song that was popular in your teen years or one played at your wedding, or one from a rock concert, movie or play you enjoyed.

- Listen to soothing notes

  Classical music in particular has been shown to slow your pulse and reduce stress hormones. In addition, it tends to increase dopamine, a brain chemical that fosters the feeling of pleasure. One possibility: "Caribbean Blue" by Enya.

- Sing a song

  Terrible singer? Doesn't matter. Singing releases endorphins and oxytocin, which relieve stress and anxiety and increase our feelings of pleasure (regardless of those sour notes). It also stimulates the parasympathetic nervous system that helps control our relaxation response.

  Don't know the lyrics? Not important. You'll still derive the same benefits. So just fumble through as best you can.

* * *

START MOVING

Sometimes simply getting the body in motion is enough to break up the tension and stress. Here are a few ways to make it happen.

- Stand up and str-e-e-e-e-tch

  Tension often collects in the neck and lower back areas. It's a good idea to try stretching every 45 minutes to keep the tightness at bay by increasing circulation and promoting relaxation.

While any stretching is better than none, next come a few especially effective routines to try.

- Cat-Cow pose

  Sit on the edge of a chair. Focus on your breathing for a few seconds. Exhale, contracting your abdominal muscles as you lean forward and round your spine. Look toward your thighs or stomach. Inhale, lifting your chest and rib cage to extend and stretch out your spine. Repeat several times.

- Basic neck stretches

  The neck has six ranges of motions. For best results, carefully stretch your neck in each of the six ranges for 15 seconds each. Alternately, you could stretch only the ranges that are feeling tight. Begin by sitting up straight in a chair. Grasp the seat of the chair with both hands.

-- Neck flexion (chin to chest): Slowly lower your neck by lowering your   chin down to your chest and hold.

-- Neck extension (leaning head back): Drop your head back as far as you can and hold.

-- Right lateral flexion (ear to shoulder): Lower your right ear toward your right shoulder and hold.

-- Left lateral flexion (ear to shoulder): Lower your left ear toward your left shoulder and hold.

-- Right rotation (chin to shoulder): Slowly turn your head to the right, aligning your chin in the direction of your right shoulder, and hold.

-- Left rotation (chin to shoulder): Slowly turn your head to the left, aligning your chin in the direction of your left shoulder, and hold.

Repeat any or all as needed.

- Shoulder shrugs

Shrug your shoulders by lifting them up toward your ears and hold tightly for 2-3 seconds. While still holding tightly, rotate your shoulders back (feeling a stretch in the chest muscles) and then let them relax them into the normal position. Do approximately ten repetitions.

Another option is to shrug your shoulders toward your ears, then simply let go and relax all the muscles from your neck down, including shoulders, chest and upper back, while saying *Ah-h-h-h*.

- Upper back stretch

    Stretch your arms out in front of you and rotate your hands thumbs down so your palms face away from each other or thumbs up so your palms face each other, depending on which is more comfortable. Next, bend over as though diving off a diving board while flexing your head (chin to chest).

    Come back up for air and repeat as needed.

Chapter Six

ONE-TOUCH RELAXATION

This technique is one of the simplest and fastest ways to relax and de-stress on the spot. Using gentle fingertip pressure on key muscles can quickly release tension throughout the body. After going through some short exercises, you could eventually be able to simply touch a particular area to elicit an immediate relaxation response.

> To begin, place your fingertips on your jaw joints right in front of your ears. Inhale while tensing your jaw muscles, bringing the upper and lower jaws together as in clenching your teeth, and hold for five seconds. Exhale and let your jaw muscles and tongue totally relax as your lower jaw drops and you release all tension while thinking *Relax*. Sense the difference between the tension and relaxation modes.

> Now repeat the exercise but using only half the tension in your jaw muscles. Repeat, using only one-fourth the tension, then finally one-eighth. At this point, it will be more difficult to sense the difference between tension and relaxation. The

objective is to set a sensory cue for relaxation through touch. You begin associating pressure from your fingertips on your jaw muscles with the desired release of tension.

Next, take a deep breath while pressing your fingertips against your jaw, then exhale while relaxing the muscles so your jaw slackens as you say *Ah-h-h-h* either aloud or silently. Your tongue should relax and fall to the base of your mouth, with the tip lightly touching the lower front teeth. Try to breathe out all tension and worry.

You can use this technique for any other areas of your body you feel tensing up at any time. With practice, you may find you can use a single touch to trigger a wave of relaxation in a particular area. You'll likely even feel the tension spreading farther—for instance, relaxing not only your jaw but also neck and shoulders.

Yeah, you got the magic touch, all right.

Chapter Seven

MEDITATION

Meditation, or mindfulness, can be a powerful way to relieve stress. Stopping to meditate for even five minutes can make a difference, and it's possible to do it anywhere—although in the driver's seat of a moving vehicle may not be the best place.

Simply clear your mind and let your thoughts run free. This can get your attention refocused while eliminating those chaotic or muddled notions that may have taken over the gray matter.

Or just focus on your breathing. Deep breathing in particular tends to slow the heart rate and lower blood pressure. All meditation uses controlled breathing, which helps your body and mind relax.

A bonus is that the benefits of meditation don't necessarily end with the session and can make it easier for you to carry on calmly throughout the rest of the day.

Your mind will probably wander during the process. This is normal, even for those who have been practicing the art for years. Just bring your thoughts back to what you were focusing on when starting your meditation—an object, your breathing or a feeling.

Remember, there is no "right" way to meditate. Stressing out about how you're breathing or what you're thinking about or whether you're doing it correctly kind of defeats the purpose. Meditation is all about taking a few moments to relax, unwind and de-stress. A five-minute meditation is a simple way to reduce stress, tension and anxiety quickly. You'll likely feel more energetic, calm and peaceful. Nice.

Some additional meditation tips:

- When possible, meditate in a quiet room where you won't be disturbed.

- Try lying on your back, if convenient. Or sitting in a chair. The idea is to make yourself as comfortable as possible.

- Meditating with your eyes closed makes it easier to stay focused. Darkness also has a calming effect on the mind.

- Try to meditate a couple times per day for a minimum of five minutes per session.

- It's better to do multiple five-minute meditations than one long session that may be tiring.

- Meditating in the morning while you're still in bed gives you a fresh start to the day; meditating before going to bed at night might improve the quality of your sleep.

Now let's get started on the meditation track. Choose a method or try each to decide which you prefer:

- Focus on something. Stop all activity and try to focus on an object or image. Alternately, picture nothing but a blank screen. The goal is to free your mind from distractions that cause stress, giving your body and mind a welcome respite.

- Relax your mind and body, close your eyes, and take some deep breaths. Now concentrate on your body, visualizing it from head to toe. Inhale to a slow count of five, seeing air fill your body. Exhale to a slow count of five, releasing any tension and stress through your breath as it leaves your body.

- Say a mantra. Sit up straight with both feet on the floor and close your eyes. Focus your attention on repeating—out loud or silently—a positive mantra (e.g., *I am at peace* or *I love myself* or *All is well*). Placing one hand on your stomach, sync up the mantra with your breaths, while letting any distracting thoughts float gently away.

- Breathe deeply. This can be done lying down, sitting, standing or walking. Breathe in deeply through your nose, then out through your nose, keeping your mouth closed but relaxed. Listen to the sound your breath makes. Place your hand on your stomach, feeling it rise as you inhale and lower as you exhale. Breathe in and breathe out at regular intervals.

- Clear your mind and thoughts. To clear your mind, acknowledge the thoughts that distressed you, then let them go. Now focus on your present moment, feeling a calming energy. Constantly bring your mind back to the present moment.

- Listen to music. Special music geared toward helping the flow into meditation can be a valuable addition to your practice. You might try researching Amazon to purchase relevant CDs. A great resource for free and easy listening is YouTube (try typing "meditation music" or "meditation for letting go" into the search bar).

Research suggests a few minutes of meditation each day may actually alter the brain's neural pathways, easing anxiety and making you more resilient to stress.

Yeah, that's the ticket.

Chapter Eight

EMOTIONAL FREEDOM TECHNIQUE

Emotional Freedom Technique (EFT or Tapping), developed in the 1990s, is a type of acupressure based on the same energy meridians used in traditional acupuncture, but without the prickly necessity for needles. The basic concept: vital energy flows through your body along certain invisible paths or meridians. These meridian points are stimulated by tapping them with your fingertips while thinking or saying certain affirmations. So nix the needles and get out the finger.

EFT helps your body heal any emotional upsets to reprogram how it responds to these stressors. In fact, it's especially powerful in treating stress and anxiety, specifically targeting your amygdala and hippocampus (huh?)—the parts of your brain that assist you in determining whether or not something is a threat.

HOW TO TAP

It should only take five minutes or less to learn the basics. Then you can start tapping away.

Use the same pressure as if tapping on a table to make a gentle drumming sound. Choose the hand you will tap the points with and use it for one whole round of tapping. You might do one round of tapping with the right hand, then one with the left. Or stick with the same hand throughout all the rounds. Use the first two or three fingers of either hand to tap lightly with your fingertips. Tap about 7-9 times on each point, in order, as follows:

1. Karate chop point

> Start by tapping the karate chop point on the outer side of your hand, midway between your wrist and the base of your little finger.

2. Inside eyebrow

> Tap on the end of the eyebrow near the bridge of your nose.

3. Side of the eye

> Tap on the bone at the outside of the eye (near the outer eyebrow).

4. Under the eye

> Tap on the bone right under your eye, lining up with your pupil.

5. Under the nose

Tap on the spot between the bottom of your nose and your upper lip.

6. Chin

Tap on the indentation of your chin, between the point of your chin and your lower lip.

7. Collarbone

Tap on your collarbone, an inch or two over from the hollow of your throat.

8. Under the arm

Tap approximately four inches below the armpit. You can reach across to tap the opposite side of your body (for example, lift your left arm and use the fingers of your right hand to tap under your left arm).

9. Top of the head

Tap in the center on the top of your head.

STEP ONE: The Setup

Begin by tapping on the karate chop point. As you do, you'll repeat a phrase (called a setup statement) three times. This will help you focus on your emotional and physical feelings to assist your body in the healing process. Allow yourself to feel the accompanying emotion.

This statement typically includes a first part stating how you feel right now, followed by a statement of self-acceptance:

> *Even though I (state how you feel), I completely and deeply love and accept myself.*

For example, if you're feeling nervous about an upcoming meeting, your setup statement might be, *Even though I feel nervous about this meeting, I completely and deeply love and accept myself.*

"Even though" statements like this allow you to tune into your body-mind connection, giving the trapped negative emotional energy a focus and path toward release.

STEP TWO: The Sequence

Next, you'll tap through the various meridian points listed above, then repeat for several rounds. Each time you tap an area, say a reminder phrase. This is a shorter version of your setup statement (for example, *this meeting* or *this stress*). Keep in mind that even though you have this problem, you still love and accept yourself. (Yeah, you do. You're freakin' awesome, you.)

PUTTING THE PROCESS TOGETHER

(to be performed in order)

1. Tune into your emotions

> Where in your body do you feel the stress, and what does it feel like?

2. Rate the intensity

> Rate the intensity of the feeling on a scale of zero to ten, with zero being little or no intensity and ten being very intense. If you don't know for sure, take your best guess.

3. Say your setup statement

> Tap continuously on the karate chop point while saying your setup statement three times. If possible, say it out loud. Allow yourself to feel the emotion. (For example, you might say, *Even though I feel this stress about the upcoming meeting, I completely and deeply love and accept myself.*)

4. Tap each sequence point 7-9 times

> Restate your issue as you tap. (For example, *this meeting* or *this stress*.)
>
> Tap the points in the following order:
>
> > a--Inside eyebrow
> >
> > b--Side of the eye
> >
> > c--Under the eye
> >
> > d--Under the nose
> >
> > e--Chin
> >
> > f--Collarbone
> >
> > g--Under the arm
> >
> > h--Top of the head

5. Take a deep breath

6. Rate the intensity

> Rate the intensity of the feeling on a scale of zero to ten, with zero being little or no intensity and ten being very intense. If it's above two, repeat steps one through five.

RESULTS

After you've completed the sequence, take a deep breath and focus on your feelings. Tune into how you feel. You may well feel a subtle sense of relief.

You can repeat the tapping sequence as many times as needed to reach your comfort level.

Usually, this exercise helps give an instant sense of relief, even if not complete or long-lasting at first. You should get even better results when you start practicing EFT regularly.

Note: While there are some variations on this basic method, this gives you a good starting point. The sequence can be much more detailed and varied, for instance, but it would be better to follow along with a practitioner (such as on a blog or YouTube) before trying such on your own.

* * *

FASTER EFT

An alternative method (a newer and simpler approach) called Faster EFT might be more your cup of tea (in addition to mint or rosemary).

1. Aim. Notice where in your body you feel the problem. It's not necessary to name the emotions or feelings.

2. Tap. Use two fingers to tap the following points:

> a -- between the eyebrows

> b -- beside the eye (at the temple)

> c -- under the eye

> d -- just below the collarbone

> *While tapping, say, Let it go or It's safe to let it go.*

3. Peace. Grasp your wrist, take a deep breath, then exhale while saying *Peace* as you think of a peaceful memory.

4. Check. Go back to your problem and notice if and how it's changed. Is the intensity of the feeling different?

5. Repeat. Repeat steps two to four until the feeling or memory has been replaced by a positive memory.

Okay now. Ready—set—start tapping.

Chapter Nine

NEURO-LINGUISTIC PROGRAMMING

Neuro-linguistic programming (NLP) was developed in the early 1970s. The basic premise of NLP is that we each create our own reality through our previous and current programming, and the brain can learn healthier patterns and ways of thinking. So come on, brain.

NLP is a collection of techniques that can be used to bring about these positive effects.

Most of us lean toward one particular mode of thinking over another: visual, auditory or kinesthetic—sight, sound or touch. People processing information visually will see images in their minds when asked a question. Those processing in the auditory mode will hear sounds rather than seeing pictures. Those leaning toward kinesthetic processing are more likely to feel emotions rather than hearing or seeing things. (Probably already had a handle on that, right?)

While NLP isn't considered a cure or a magic bullet, it can help decrease stress to help you live your life in a more productive manner.

Following are several great tools you can try using to better manage that stress in your life. These tools can be easily learned and utilized even if you've never studied NLP.

- Reframing

    Reframing how you view stress can be an effective way to manage it. If you learn to reframe and harness the power of stress or anxiety, it could actually prove a steppingstone in your life.

    Like the caveman, your body is hardwired for survival—always on the lookout for that dangerous predator or the next stressful situation. In other words, a bit paranoid. The oldest part of your brain works hard to protect you, but this natural tendency to be ever-vigilant for danger and certain death can result in harmful stress.

    So how can you reframe stress? First, see it as a sign something in your life needs to be addressed or changed. Second, realize there's likely a secondary gain attached to your behaviors. This is a benefit you may derive from not overcoming a problem or challenge—a sort of payoff that isn't usually a conscious choice. For instance, putting up with a stressful job because you enjoy the sympathy when others feel sorry for you.

The key is to figure out what that payoff is so you can reframe (or view) the stress from a different perspective and change how you react to it.

- Altering the submodalities

   Submodalities, one of the easiest and most powerful NLP techniques, help you change the impact of specific memories. This works in two ways:

   1. You can make good memories better and stronger

   2. You can make bad memories weaker

   This is a relatively simple concept. Take a specific memory and change such things as how bright the colors are, how loud the sounds are or how close the image is to you. In other words, play with these various aspects of the memory's image in your mind, as though tuning a TV picture.

To make the memory stronger, make the image big and close while using vivid colors with the volume turned up; to make the memory weaker, push it into the distance while using faded colors with the volume turned down. And voila! New television show, with you as the all-powerful, but unpaid, director.

- Using relaxation anchors

  Anchors are simple to use but require some work before the stressful moment comes into play. They involve closing your eyes and thinking back to something calm and relaxing in your life. Just take a few deep, cleansing breaths and focus on a positive memory or vision, like being at the beach.

  See yourself walking along the water's edge, enjoying the feel of your feet sinking into the sand and the warm sun on your back. Listen to the gentle lapping of the waves and smell the salty sea air. Stay with that vision until you've reached a peak state of relaxation and peace. Then immediately create a physical anchor (for example, press your middle finger and your thumb together; or squeeze one hand into a fist while thinking *Relax*). Release the image and go about your normal day.

You can test the anchor by duplicating the physical action while saying *Relax* in your mind to see if you get that laid-back feeling again. If not, try going back to the beach and installing the anchor again.

You'll want to go through this process several times over a few days to create a strong anchor. It may be necessary to repeat the process periodically. When you get anxious or stressed, you can then use the anchor to bring back those positive feelings. Or just actually head to the beach.

- Imagining a thick wall

Imagine a thick wall of bricks or concrete in front of you. You can place the emotion of the stressful situation on the other side of that wall while hiding safely behind it. Quick, crouch down, out of sight.

- Turning your self-talk into Donald Duck

  Hear those annoying words inside your head spoken in the voice of Donald Duck. Hard to take it seriously now, isn't it? *Quack.*

- Changing the quality of another's talk

  Keep hearing another person's negative, irritating or judgmental voice rambling about inside your head? Imagine that person speaking in super slo-o-o-w motion. Or sounding like Kermit the frog. Maybe even throw in Miss Piggy and her porcine attitude, for good measure.

- Playing a funny song in your mind

  Tune out the stress and turn up a funny song. It could be a happy ditty you've heard on the radio, a snappy theme song from a sitcom or movie, even a few bars from a commercial. Lyrics are optional.

Chapter Ten

ODDS & ENDS

And now we come to a few odds and ends to tack onto your arsenal of stress busters. See which ones tickle your fancy.

- Try liming

  > Liming comes from the Caribbean and is the art of doing nothing, guilt free. It's taking time for personal pursuits done purely for the enjoyment of it. To partake, choose one of your favorite pleasures—be it leaning back in your chair and remembering a funny story, humming or dancing to a favorite tune, gazing out the window and letting your mind drift or whatever. The main idea is to step away from the tasks and expectations of the day and let the tension melt away. So just pretend you're in the Caribbean and enjoying a moment of lazy pleasure. It's expected, mahn.

- Organize things

Chaos in your surroundings can create stress you may be unaware of. Rearranging things re-establishes order and can get your stress level down. You may even find a stray lost sock or two.

- Discard junk

  Clutter has a way of sneaking up on us and finding ourselves buried in unnecessary stuff tends to increase our level of stress hormones. To get started, place a garbage bag front and center in the room you deem the biggest culprit. Whenever you walk by it, throw in two or more items that need to vacate the premises. No take backs.

- Start counting

  Counting gives your mind something neutral to focus on. This simple tactic can get you onto a more relaxed track. Just stay away from new math.

- Say your CBAs

  Try reciting the alphabet backward. This requires you to concentrate on the letters, so by the time you get to P-O-N, you may have forgotten what was bothering you. A backwards alphabet is tricky.

- Take a virtual vacation

  You might just reminisce about a favorite vacation you took. Or you could imagine a dream getaway. One suggestion is to close your eyes and visualize being on an ocean liner, feeling the rhythm of the waves while inhaling the fragrance of the ocean. Something to make you smile. The act of visualizing and smiling causes a release of endorphins, your natural stress relievers. Just close your eyes, let your mind go on vacation, and grin like a ninny. Almost as good as being there (sort of).

- Get out the iron

  Focusing on the repetitive back-and-forth motion across the ironing board can mimic going into a meditative state. Back and forth. Ba-a-ck and forth. Ba-a-ck ...a-a-and ...

- Brush your skin

Stroking your skin with a dry brush stimulates nerve endings. This will activate the parasympathetic nervous system, triggering a relaxed response. And it just feels good.

- Massage yourself

  Find the part of your body that feels tight and knead away the tension. Afterwards, finish with a full body shake. Not as satisfying as a professional massage, but cheaper.

- Kiss someone

  This one is easier with a partner. It's been noted that kissing can relieve stress by creating a sense of connectedness, releasing those feel-good endorphins. So go ahead; take a breath mint, pucker up and enjoy.

- Scream at something

  But not someone. Inanimate objects are less likely to fight back. Since stress can build up in us if we don't release any of it, there's nothing more satisfying than a good old primal scream to push negativity out of our system. This releases endorphins to provide a natural source of relief. If others are nearby, though, you might want to shout into a pillow to save face. This will also prevent harming another's eardrums or feelings.

- Laugh hard

  As in good, old-fashioned belly laugh. Har-har-harring reduces the levels of epinephrine, cortisol and other stress hormones. And the best part is you don't have to wait for something funny to tickle your innards. What counts is the physical act of laughing. So just start laughing (though you may prefer to be alone for this to preserve your reputation as one of the sane).

- Heave a sigh

  A good, heartfelt sigh can feel like taking a huge weight off your shoulders because it requires you to lower them. At the same time, it makes you relax your jaw and release tension in your upper body. And presto—you find yourself in a more relaxed state.

- Lighten up

  Get out in the sun. As your body absorbs sunlight, mood-stabilizing chemicals like serotonin shoot up. Park at the far end of the lot, take a stroll down the block, throw open the curtains at home. Soak up those golden rays.

- Sniff an orange

  Inhaling the scent of an orange can significantly reduce your stress levels. Slice up an orange and breathe in the refreshing aroma or try a whiff of orange essential oil.

- Pet a pet

  Get your hands on a friendly cat or furry dog and start petting. Stroking a pet can trigger the release of oxytocin to reduce your cortisol level. And it's also nice for the little critter.

- Take a stroll

  Try changing the scene. Step outside and take a lap around the house or a quick hike down the street and back. While out, focus on the sights and sounds in the area. Let your mind relax and enjoy.

- Float away

  Imagine you're floating in the air, drifting to the ground like a falling leaf or feather. Feel the slow and gentle descent, with nothing but air touching you. Relax into the peace and quiet. Have a soft landing.

Admit it. We're feeling better now, aren't we? Just a little?

Chapter Eleven

BONUS TIP

And finally, the number one way to lower stress: Having an "attitude of gratitude."

This one concept can not only make you healthier, it can also make life more fun and pleasurable.

Researchers at the University of California recently found people who take time each day to focus on what they're grateful for produce an average of 23 percent less cortisol. So stop for a few short moments or long minutes to think about all the great things present in your life. Every day. Several times a day.

To get the ball rolling, consider the following:

If the population of the world was broken down into only 100 people:

> 80 would live in substandard housing (i.e. no running water or electricity, etc.)

> 50 would be malnourished, living off perhaps one small meal a day

> 70 would be unable to read

In addition, here's a partial list of what we might each be grateful for every day. Pause briefly to consider each listing and how the lack of it would affect our lives. Feel free to add your own hundreds of points of gratitude.

1. Being alive (oh, yeah—número uno)

2. Sense of sight

3. Sense of hearing

4. Houses

5. Electricity

6. Copy machines

7. Safety pins

8. Elevators

9. Staples

10. Clean water to drink

11. Coffee to wake up and smell

12. Pets

13. Pooper scoopers

14. Glue

15. The ability to read

16. Books

17. Beds

18. Bicycles

19. Garbage pickup

20. Ladders

21. Freedom of speech

22. Sticky notes

23. Scissors

24. Indoor plumbing

25. Sense of taste

26. Paper

27. Pens and pencils

28. Erasers and Wite-Out

29. Air conditioning

30. Grocery stores

31. Music

32. Buttons

33. Paper clips

34. Movies

35. Central heating

36. Pots and pans

37. Computers

38. Buckets

39. Windows

40. Flashlights

41. Calendars

42. Honeybees

43. Combs

44. Mistakes to learn from

45. Works of art

46. Printers

47. Toothbrushes

48. Sunglasses

49. Measuring spoons

50. Photographs

51. Ready-made clothing

52. Razors

53. Chocolate

54. Chocolate-covered anything

55. Mirrors

56. Vacuum cleaners

57. Refrigerators

58. Thunderstorms

59. Lightning

60. Lightning rods

61. Blacktop streets

62. Concrete sidewalks

63. Facial tissues

64. Napkins

65. Wastebaskets

66. Dish soap

67. Paper plates

68. Tables

69. Chairs

70. Snow

71. Snow shovels

72. Forks

73. Hammers

74. Lightbulbs

75. Ice cubes

76. Maps

77. Traffic signals

78. Cameras

79. Restaurants

80. Cups

81. Hot showers on cold days

82. Hot showers on hot days

83. Mountains

84. Blinds and drapes

85. Door locks

86. Fans

87. Eyeglasses

88. Paint

89. Paint remover

90. Matches

91. Firefighters

92. Zippers

93. Planes

94. Trains

95. Automobiles

96. Rain on a warm summer night

97. Laughter

98. Waking up today

99. Life's challenges—for helping us grow and become who we are

And of course (drumroll, please) ...

100. You—for being who you are and working to become the best version of yourself

Chapter Twelve

WRAPPING UP

Stop catastrophizing!

When stress sets in and anxiety is the order of the day, it's easy to get into a mindset known as "catastrophic thinking" or "catastrophizing." Left to its own devices, your mind goes rogue and latches onto the gloomiest and darkest of thoughts. Egads, the horror! What if, in your wildest imagination, things go horrendously, unbearably wrong? What if the very worst of your fears actually happens? What if your world collapses and the Earth explodes into a gazillion tiny pieces? Then what will you do?

Before your own world and the Earth disappear forever, try taking a few deep breaths and consider how likely it is the very worst will happen. Chances are the outcome for your particular worry won't be as bad as you're imagining. And even if it is—well, most likely the Earth is still intact and circling the sun, so it could still be worse.

We've taken a serious look at the effects of stress, gone over several remedies you can try out and in the process had some fun. Once you've taken that deep breath, please go back over the previous material and choose a favorite way of coping. You might, in fact, choose several favorites. So dig in, get going and DE-STRESS.

Cheers!

Please leave a rating for this book on Amazon. Thank you!

RESOURCE GUIDE

(in addition to your own Google searches)

Chapter One

For a guided breathing process, visit:
www.5minutemeditation.com

Chapter Three

Where to buy essential oils:

DoTERRA:
www.doTERRA.com

Young Living:
www.youngliving.com

Chapter Four

Where to buy CBD Oil:
www.cbdoilusers.com/cbd-oil-reviews/
www.bestcbdoils.org/best-companies/

Chapter Eight

For more information on EFT, visit:
www.eft.mercola.com

For more information on Faster EFT, visit:
www.fastereft.com

For videos on various topics presented in the book, visit:

www.YouTube.com

APPENDIX

SIGNS AND SYMPTOMS OF STRESS

The following are a few of the health issues associated with chronic stress, starting with common signs and leading into more serious potential long-term effects.

- Strange and/or recurring dreams

    Having wild and crazy dreams or any one particular dream night after night could be a warning sign that you're feeling stressed. Such dreams can take a toll on you both mentally and physically, making you feel tired, draggy and oh so edgy. YES, I SAID EDGY. Uh ... ahem.

- Sleep issues

    Most people experience a sleepless night here and there due to stress caused by family problems, work or financial issues, etc. Waking up at night with difficulty getting back to sleep further impacts one's ability to handle the stress of the day.

- Hair loss

  Stress can put your hair follicles into a resting stage, resulting in strands of hair falling out a few months later. Fortunately, this tends to be a temporary condition, so don't throw away your stylist's number.

- Tooth and jaw pain

  You may manage to keep a lid on stress during the day, but during the night your subconscious takes over and shows who's boss (it's the subconscious). That's when you might start grinding your pearly whites, leading to sore gums, jaw and/or mouth. Not a fair way to deal with stress. After all, it's not like your mouth ever did anything to get you in trouble.

- Stomach and gastrointestinal problems

  Stress seems to affect the gastrointestinal system like it affects the brain, causing that butterfly feeling in our stomach when we're nervous. The flight or fight response in the central nervous system can even shut down digestion. If you're constantly stressed, this can lead to stomachaches, diarrhea, irritable bowel syndrome, ulcers and food allergies. Yeah, we're talking fun stuff here.

- Common illnesses

  Worry and tension can lower the immune system, making you more susceptible to illnesses like the common cold or flu. If you find yourself getting sick more than the average person, catching every virus that comes loping into town, the real culprit could be stress.

  Under stress, the body releases cortisol, the hormone that affects the inflammatory response to fight off whatever is causing the discomfort. As the immune cells become less sensitive to cortisol, they're unable to regulate the needed response. Then comes exposure to a virus—and *Hey there, cold or flu.*

- Abdominal fat

  Medical professionals have suspected for some years that chronic stress may be a contributing factor for abdominal fat. One reason is that stress often causes us to reach for carb-heavy foods (cue the bread and cake and cookies) that increase the body's serotonin level, making us feel oh-so better. This positive effect encourages us to continue the cycle. The result? Loss of muscle mass and softer belly.

- Fatigue

  Of course, we all get tired on occasion. But if you're feeling constantly fatigued, there's likely more to it. Fatigue can be a symptom of stress, especially if you're having trouble sleeping.

- Back pain

  You might experience back pain when you're stressed out because the body instinctively pumps out hormones when in fight or flight mode. That raises your blood pressure and heart rate, tightening muscles and increasing pain. It can even trigger painful muscle spasms and cries of *Oh, my aching back.*

- Headaches

Stress can trigger a tension headache. No surprise there. One survey found the majority of military service members at a headache clinic attributed their pain to stress, with other common causes cited as lack of sleep, alcohol, dehydration. And being in the service.

- Mood swings and depression

  Experiencing stress on a chronic basis contributes to a variety of changes in the brain. Yes, that might be good for some people, but we're talking a possible imbalance of positive neurotransmitters like serotonin and dopamine. These imbalances can negatively affect mood, appetite, sleep and libido. Besides making us feel irritable, depressed or angry, this can also lead to feeling helpless, overwhelmed and out of control. And what's the fun in that?

- Aging

  Chronic stress affects processes within the body that work to keep skin looking young and healthy. Stress can allow toxins to cross the blood-brain barrier and negatively impact aging. High cortisol levels have been shown to reduce the size of the hippocampus, and the progression of Alzheimer's disease may be linked to the size of this area. Stress also inhibits the regeneration of new blood cells, which can age a person both psychologically and physically. There's just no win there.

- Heart problems

  Yeah, getting even more serious now. Chronic stress causes inflammation that may damage blood vessels, increasing the risk of hypertension, atherosclerosis and stroke. It restricts the arteries and thickens the blood, forcing the heart to work harder, and can also cause a surplus of disease-fighting white blood cells that leads to hardening of the arteries.

  Whoa, this is stressing me out.

- Diabetes

  Stress doesn't necessarily cause diabetes, but it can make it worse since stress hormones in your body may directly affect glucose levels. Mental stress in people with type 2 diabetes can cause an increase in blood sugar levels, while physical stress can cause an increase in these levels for people with either type 1 or type 2 diabetes.

- Dementia and cognitive impairment

    Although research hasn't yet proven conclusive, there are some logical reasons why stress could be linked to dementia. One is that stress compromises the body's immune system, known to play an important role in the development of dementia. Another is the strong connection between stress and depression, the latter associated with a more rapid decline in thinking skills. In addition, stress has negative effects on learning and memory since it kills brain cells.

    Furthermore ... uh, furthermore ... Wait, what was I saying?

- Addiction

    Stress can cause behavioral changes that could lead to addiction as a coping mechanism. People with chronic stress might turn to alcohol, drugs or excessive eating, temporarily raising their serotonin and dopamine levels that help them feel good. But these elevated hormonal levels will run out in short order, leaving the person feeling worse than before and craving a path to feeling good again. And the cycle continues.

Stress could also cause an increase in addictions like gambling, watching television or playing video games instead of dealing with the stress in a healthier manner.

Now, where did I put that remote?

Okay, enough with the stressful indicators. We all get the idea, right? But now we have many tools to choose from to deal with this issue.

Best of luck!

Please leave a rating for this book on Amazon. Thank you!

NOTES